DOSAGE CALCULATIONS FOR NURSING

THINGS YOU SHOULD KNOW
(QUESTIONS AND ANSWERS)

Rumi Michael Leigh

Introduction

I would like to thank and congratulate you for purchasing this book, " *Dosage calculations for nursing, things you should know (questions and answers)*" series.

This book will help you understand, revise and have a good general knowledge and keywords of dosage calculations.

Thanks again for purchasing this book, I hope you enjoy it!

Table of Contents

Introduction	*2*
Chapter 1: conversions	*4*
Chapter 2: ounce to mL	*6*
Chapter 3: milligram to microgram	*8*
Chapter 4: teaspoons to milliliters	*10*
Chapter 5: grams to microgram	*12*
Chapter 6: dosage calculations: part 1	*15*
Chapter 6: dosage calculations: part 2	*20*
Conclusion	*26*

Chapter 1: conversions

1) 1 milliliter (mL) =? cubic centimeter(cc)
- 1mL = 1cc
2) 1 liter (L) =? milliliters(mL)
- 1L = 1000mL
3) 1 milligram (mg) =? microgram(mcg)
- 1mg = 1000mcg
4) 1 gram (g) =? milligrams(mg)
- 1g = 1000mg
5) 1 kilogram (1kg) =? grams(g)
- 1kg = 1000g
6) 1 kilogram (kg) =? pounds
- 1kg = 2.2 pounds
7) 1 ounce (oz) =? milliliters(mL)
- 1oz = 30 mL
8) 1 teaspoon =? milliliters(mL)
- 1 teaspoon = 5 mL
9) 1 tablespoon =? teaspoons
- 1 tablespoon = 3 teaspoons

10) 1 tablespoon =? milliliters(mL)
- 1 tablespoon = 15 mL
11) 1 ounce (oz) =? tablespoons
- 1oz = 2 tablespoons
12) 1 mL =? drops
- 1 mL = 20 drops
13) 1 mL of blood =? drops
- 1 mL of blood = 15 drops
14) 1 mL of Buretrol =? drops
- 1 mL of Buretrol = 60 microdrops

Chapter 2: ounce to mL

1) 360 ounces equals how many mL?
- If 1 oz = 30 mL
- then 360 oz = 360 x 30 = 10800mL

2) 320 ounces equals how many mL?
- If 1 oz = 30 mL
- then 320 oz = 320 x 30 = 9600mL

3) 180 ounces equals how many mL?
- If 1 oz = 30 mL
- then 180 oz = 180 x 30 = 5400mL

4) 120 ounces equals how many mL?
- If 1 oz = 30 mL
- then 120 oz = 120 x 30 = 3600mL

5) 80 ounces equals how many mL?
- If 1 oz = 30 mL
- then 80 oz = 80 x 30 = 2400mL

6) 70 ounces equals how many mL?
- If 1 oz = 30 mL
- then 70 oz = 70 x 30 = 2100mL

7) 60 ounces equals how many mL?
- If 1 oz = 30 mL
- then 60 oz = 60 x 30 = 1800mL

8) 45 ounces equals how many mL?
- If 1 oz = 30 mL
- then 45 oz = 45 x 30 = 1350ml

9) 30 ounces equals how many mL?
- If 1 oz = 30 mL
- then 30 oz = 360 x 30 = 900mL

10) 15 ounces equals how many mL?
- If 1 oz = 30 mL
- then 15 oz = 15 x 30 = 450mL

Chapter 3: milligram to microgram

1) 10 milligrams equals how many microgram?
- If 1mg = 1,000 mcg
- then 10 mg = 10 x 1000 mcg = 10000 mcg

2) 25 milligrams equals how many microgram?
- If 1mg = 1,000 mcg
- then 25 mg = 25 x 1000 mcg = 25000 mcg

3) 35 milligrams equals how many microgram?
- If 1mg = 1,000 mcg
- then 35 mg = 35 x 1000 mcg = 35000 mcg

4) 40 milligrams equals how many microgram?
- If 1mg = 1,000 mcg
- then 40 mg = 40 x 1000 mcg = 40000 mcg

5) 46 milligrams equals how many microgram?
- If 1mg = 1,000 mcg
- then 46 mg = 46 x 1000 mcg = 46000 mcg

6) 48 milligrams equals how many microgram?
- If 1mg = 1,000 mcg
- then 48 mg = 48 x 1000 mcg = 48000 mcg

7) 52 milligrams equals how many microgram?
- If 1mg = 1,000 mcg
- then 52 mg = 52 x 1000 mcg = 52000 mcg

8) 60 milligrams equals how many microgram?
- If 1mg = 1,000 mcg
- then 60 mg = 60 x 1000 mcg = 60000 mcg

9) 75 milligrams equals how many microgram?
- If 1mg = 1,000 mcg
- then 75 mg = 75 x 1000 mcg = 75000 mcg

10) 80 milligrams equals how many microgram?
- If 1mg = 1,000 mcg
- then 80 mg = 80 x 1000 mcg = 80000 mcg

Chapter 4: teaspoons to milliliters

1) 12 teaspoons equals how many milliliters?
- If 1 teaspoon = 5 mL
- then 12 teaspoons = 12 x 5 mL = 60 mL

2) 15 teaspoons equals how many milliliters?
- If 1 teaspoon = 5 mL
- then 15 teaspoons = 15 x 5 mL = 75 mL

3) 18 teaspoons equals how many milliliters?
- If 1 teaspoon = 5 mL
- then 18 teaspoons = 18 x 5 mL = 90 mL

4) 25 teaspoons equals how many milliliters?
- If 1 teaspoon = 5 mL
- then 25 teaspoons = 25 x 5 mL = 125 mL

5) 29 teaspoons equals how many milliliters?
- If 1 teaspoon = 5 mL
- then 29 teaspoons = 29 x 5 mL = 145 mL

6) 32 teaspoons equals how many milliliters?
- If 1 teaspoon = 5 mL
- then 32 teaspoons = 32 x 5 mL = 160 mL

7) 35 teaspoons equals how many milliliters?
- If 1 teaspoon = 5 mL
- then 35 teaspoons = 35 x 5 mL = 175 mL

8) 40 teaspoons equals how many milliliters?
- If 1 teaspoon = 5 mL
- then 40 teaspoons = 40 x 5 mL = 200 mL

9) 45 teaspoons equals how many milliliters?
- If 1 teaspoon = 5 mL
- then 45 teaspoons = 45 x 5 mL = 225 mL

10) 50 teaspoons equals how many milliliters?
- If 1 teaspoon = 5 mL
- then 50 teaspoons = 50 x 5 mL = 250 mL

Chapter 5: grams to microgram

1) 0.15 gram equals how many micrograms?
   - 1 g = 1000 mg, then 0.15 g = 150 mg
   - if 1 mg = 1000 mcg, then 150 mg = 150 x 1,000 mcg = 150,000 mcg
2) 0.25 gram equals how many micrograms?
   - 1 g = 1000 mg, then 0.25 g = 250 mg
   - if 1 mg = 1000 mcg, then 250 mg = 250 x 1,000 mcg = 250,000 mcg
3) 0.55 gram equals how many micrograms?
   - 1 g = 1000 mg, then 0.55 g = 550 mg
   - if 1 mg = 1000 mcg, then 550 mg = 550 x 1,000 mcg = 550,000 mcg
4) 0.6 gram equals how many micrograms?
   - 1 g = 1000 mg, then 0.6 g = 600 mg

- if 1 mg = 1000 mcg, then 600 mg = 600 x 1,000 mcg = 600,000 mcg
5) 0.75 gram equals how many micrograms?
- 1 g = 1000 mg, then 0.75 g = 750 mg
- if 1 mg = 1000 mcg, then 750 mg = 750 x 1,000 mcg = 750,000 mcg
6) 0.8 gram equals how many micrograms?
- 1 g = 1000 mg, then 0.8 g = 800 mg
- if 1 mg = 1000 mcg, then 800 mg = 800 x 1,000 mcg = 800,000 mcg
7) 0.9 gram equals how many micrograms?
- 1 g = 1000 mg, then 0.9 g = 900 mg
- if 1 mg = 1000 mcg, then 900 mg = 900 x 1,000 mcg = 900,000 mcg
8) 0.95 gram equals how many micrograms?
- 1 g = 1000 mg, then 0.95 g = 950 mg
- if 1 mg = 1000 mcg, then 950 mg = 950 x 1,000 mcg = 950,000 mcg
9) 2 grams equals how many micrograms?
- 1 g = 1000 mg, then 2 g = 2000 mg
- if 1 mg = 1000 mcg, then 2000 mg = 2000 x 1,000 mcg = 2000000 mcg
10) 2.5 grams equals how many micrograms?

- 1 g = 1000 mg, then 2.5 g = 2500 mg
- if 1 mg = 1000 mcg, then 2500 mg = 2500 x 1,000 mcg = 2500000 mcg

Chapter 6: dosage calculations: part 1

1) A doctor's order for an intravenous medication is 2 mg. The vial contains 0.8 mg/mL. How many mL is necessary to administer the medication?
   - 0.8 mg = 1 mL
   - 2 mg = (2 mg/0.8 mg) x 1 mL = 2.5 mL
   - So, 2.5 mL is necessary to administer the medication.
2) The doctor's order says to infuse 3 L of normal saline at 200 mL/h. If the infusion was started at 07:00 in the morning, at what time will the infusion be complete?
   - 3 L = 3,000 mL
   - if 250 mL = 1h, so 3,000 mL = (3,000mL/200mL) x 1h = 15h
   - 07:00 + 15h = 22h

- So, the infusion will be complete at 10:00 in the evening.
3) According to the doctor's prescription, you must inject 200 mg of medicine B intramuscularly. What quantity in mL of medicine B should you prepare knowing that a vial of this medicine contains 2 mL at 60 mg/mL?
   - 1 mL = 60 mg, so 2 mL = 120 mg
   - So, 2 mL vial of medicine B contains 120 mg
   - 120 mg = 2 mL of medicine B, so 200 mg = 200/120 x 2 mL = 3.33 mL of medicine B
   - So, 3.33 mL of medicine B should be prepared.
4) A 65 kg patient should receive 0.1 mg/kg. There are vial of 1 mg/mL. How many mL should be administered?
   - 1 kg = 0.1 mg, so 65 kg = 65 x 0.1 mg = 6.5 mg
   - If 1 mg = 1 mL, 6.5 mg = 6.5 mL
   - So, 6.5 mL should be administered.
5) A 55 kg patient should receive 0.5 mg/kg. There are vial of 2 mg/mL. How many mL should be administered?
   - 1 kg = 0.5 mg, so 55 kg = 55 x 0.5 mg = 27.5 mg

- If 2 mg = 1 mL, 27.5 mg = (27.5/2) x 1 mL = 13.75 mL
- So, 13.75 mL should be administered.

6) A client receives an intravenous saline infusion of 2 liters over 24 hours. Calculate the flow rate in mL/h and drops/min.
    - Flow rate = volume (mL)/time (h) = 2000 mL/ 24 h = 83.33 mL/h
    - 1 mL of intravenous saline = 20 drops
    - 2000 mL of intravenous saline = 2000 mL x 20 drops = 40,000 drops
    - Flow rate = volume (drops)/time (minute) = 40,000 drops/24 x 60 minutes = 27.78 drops/minute
    - So, the flow rate = 83.33 mL/h or 27.78 drops/minute

7) What is the flow rate in drops/min if the prescription is to transfuse 400 mL of blood in 3 hours?
    - Flow rate = volume (drops)/time (minute)
    - time = (3 x 60) minutes
    - 1 mL = 15 drops, so 400 mL = 400 x 15 drops = 6000 drops

- Flow rate = 6000 drops/(3 x 60) minute = 33.33 drops/minute
- So, the flow rate in drops/min is 33.33 drops/minute

8) You must administer an IV antibiotic dissolved in 100 mL of liquid over 45 minutes. What is the flow rate with a Buretrol system?
    - 1 mL = 60 microdrops
    - So, 100 mL = 100 x 60 microdrops = 6,000 microdrops
    - Flow rate = microdrops/minute = 6000 microdrops/45 minutes = 133.33 microdrops/minute
    - So, the flow rate is 133.33 microdrops/minute

9) According to the doctor's prescription, the nurse must dilute 40 mL of antibiotic in 60 mL of 0.9% of NaCl. Everything is administered by infusion over 30 minutes using a Buretrol device. Calculate the infusion rate in microdrops/min.
    - 1 mL = 60 microdrops
    - 100 mL = 100 x 60 microdrops = 6,000 microdrops
    - Infusion rate = volume (microdrops)/time (minute) = 6,000/30 = 200 microdrops/minute

- So, the flow rate is 200 microdrops/minute
10) When you arrive at 08:00 in the morning, there are 450 mL left in the 0.9% of NaCl infusion bag. The infusion should be finished by 11 am. Calculate the infusion rate in mL/h.
    - 08:30 to 10:00 = 2 hours 30 minutes or 150 mins or 2.5 hours
    - Infusion rate = Volume (mL)/time(h) = 450 mL /2.5 hours = 180 mL/h
    - So, the infusion rate is 180 mL/h

Chapter 6: dosage calculations: part 2

1) An intravenous infusion runs at 25 drops/min. After how long in hours and minutes will the patient have received 10 dl?
   - 10 dl = 1000 mL
   - If 1 mL = 20 drops, 1000 mL = 1000 mL x 20 drops = 20,000 drops
   - 25 drops = 1 min, then 20,000 drops = 20,000/25 x 1 min = 800 minutes = 13.33 hours
   - So, the patient will have received 10 dl in approximately 13h 20 minutes
2) An intravenous infusion flows at a rate of 12 drops/min. It should be administered in 5 hours. Calculate the volume in mL to be infused.
   - 5 hours = 300 minutes
   - Flow rate = 12 drops/min

- 1 mL = 20 drops
- 12 drops = 12/20 x 1 mL = 0.6 mL
- So, flow rate = 0.6 mL/min
- If 1 min = 0.6 mL, then 300 minutes = 300 x 0.6 mL = 180 mL
- So, the volume in mL to be infused is 180 mL

3) You have 2 liters of 20% of medicine A. How many mg/mL of medicine A do you have?
    - 2 liters = 2000 mL
    - 1% → 1 g → 100 mL
    - 1% → 1000 mg → 100 mL
    - 20% → 20,000 mg → 100 mL
    - 100 mL = 20,000 mg,
    - So, 2000 mL = 2000/100 x 20,000 mg = 400,000 mg
    - 400,000 mg/2000 mL
    - So, you have 200mg/mL

4) You have 1 liter of 50% of medicine B. How many mg/mL of medicine B do you have?
    - 1 liter = 1000 mL
    - 1% → 1 g → 100 mL
    - 1% → 1000 mg → 100 mL
    - 50% ☐ 50,000 mg ☐ 100 mL

- 100 mL = 50,000 mg,
- So, 1000 mL = 1000/100 x 50,000 mg = 500,000 mg
- 500,000 mg/1000 mL
- So, you have 500mg/mL

5) 200 mg of medicine B contained in a 4 mL vial is diluted with 6 mL of solvent. What is the percentage of the solution?
   - 200 mg = 0.2 g
   - Volume = 4mL + 6mL = 10 mL
   - Concentration = mass/volume = g/mL = 0.2 g/10 mL
   - 10 x C = 0.2 x 100
   - Concentration = 2%

6) 300 mg of medicine Y contained in a 5 mL vial is diluted with 10 mL of solvent. What is the percentage of the solution?
   - We are looking for the concentration % of the solution.
   - 300 mg = 0.3 g
   - Volume = 5mL +10mL = 15 mL
   - Concentration = mass/volume = g/mL = 0.3 g/15 mL

- 15 x C = 0.3 x 100
- Concentration = 2%

7) 150 mg of medicine A contained in a 2 mL vial is diluted with 8 mL of solvent. What is the percentage of the solution?
   - We are looking for the concentration % of the solution.
   - 150 mg = 0.15 g
   - Volume = 2mL + 8mL = 10 mL
   - Concentration = mass/volume = g/mL = 0.15 g/10 mL
   - 10 x C = 0.15 x 100
   - Concentration = 1.5%

8) You add a 2 mL vial of medicine A dosed at 80 mg/mL into a syringe containing 5 mL of 0.9% of NaCl. What is the concentration in % of the solution obtained?
   - 1 mL of medicine A = 80 mg, so 2 mL of medicine A = 160 mg
   - 160 mg = 0.16 g
   - Volume = 2 mL + 5 mL = 7 mL
   - Concentration = mass/volume = g/mL = 0.16 g/15 mL
   - 7 x C = 0.16 x 100

- Concentration = 2.29%

9) You add a 3 mL vial of medicine B dosed at 60 mg/mL into a syringe containing 7 mL of 0.9% of NaCl. What is the concentration in % of the solution obtained?
   - 1 mL of medicine A = 60 mg, so 3 mL of medicine A = 180 mg
   - 180 mg = 0.18 g
   - Volume = 3 mL + 7 mL = 10 mL
   - Concentration = mass/volume = g/mL = 0.18 g/10 mL
   - 10 x C = 0.18 x 100
   - Concentration = 1.8%

10) A patient should receive 25 g of medicine B intravenously. You have vials of 90% of medicine B available. How many mL do you withdraw from the vial to prepare the infusion?
    - 1% → 1 g → 100 mL
    - 90% → 90 g → 100 mL
    - 90 g = 100 mL, so 25 g = 25/90 x 100 mL = 27.77 mL

11) Mister Johnson should receive 45 g of medicine Z intravenously. You have vials of 75% of medicine Z

available. How many mL do you withdraw from the vial to prepare the infusion?

- 1% → 1 g → 100 mL
- 75% → 75 g → 100 mL
- 75 g = 100 mL, so 45 g = 45/75 x 100 mL = 60 mL

12) Madame Sarah should receive 35 g of medicine A intravenously. You have vials of 80% of medicine A available. How many mL do you withdraw from the vial to prepare the infusion?

- 1% → 1 g → 100 mL
- 80% → 80 g → 100 mL
- 80 g = 100 mL, so 35 g = 35/80 x 100 mL = 43.75 mL

Conclusion

Thank you again for purchasing this book. I hope it has helped you in your journey to understanding dosage calculations for nursing.

Please, if you enjoyed this book, I would like you to leave a review. It'd be appreciated.

Thank you.

www.ingramcontent.com/pod-product-compliance
Lightning Source LLC
Chambersburg PA
CBHW050328220526
45465CB00005B/2175